HOLISTIC APPROACHES TO HOLISTIC MANAGING PANCREATIC DISORDER

Holistic Odyssey to Managing Pancreatic Disorders through Integrative Wellness Strategies

DR. CHRIS FRIEDRICH

CHAPTER ONE **15**

UNDERSTANDING PANCREATIC DISORDERS 15

CHAPTER TWO **20**

HOLISTIC APPROACH TO HEALTH 20

CHAPTER THREE **27**

NUTRITION AND PANCREATIC HEALTH 27

CHAPTER FOUR **31**

LINK BETWEEN MIND AND BODY 31

CHAPTER FIVE **34**

HERBAL REMEDIES AND ADVANCED THERAPIES............................34

CHAPTER SIX **38**

MODIFICATIONS TO LIFESTYLE FOR PANCREATIC HEALTH..............38

CHAPTER SEVEN **46**

INTEGRATING CONVENTIONAL AND HOLISTIC APPROACHES 46

CHAPTER EIGHT..**51**

SELF-CARE AND PATIENT EMPOWERMENT....................................51

CHAPTER NINE **57**

MEAL PLANS AND RECIPES 57

CHAPTER TEN **61**

PROSPECTS FOR PANCREATIC HEALTH IN THE FUTURE...................61

CONCLUSION 64

Disclaimer

This book on Herbal Remedies is intended solely for informational and educational purposes.

The content provided within this book is based on general knowledge and should not be considered as professional advice. The author is not a licensed medical professional, and the information presented here is not intended to diagnose, treat, cure, or prevent any disease.

Readers are advised to consult with qualified healthcare professionals before initiating any herbal remedies or making changes to their existing health regimen. The author and publisher disclaim any responsibility for any adverse effects or consequences resulting from the use of information contained in this book.

It's important to note that the content of this book is not endorsed by any specific platform or affiliated with any product or service.

The author does not receive any compensation or benefits from the promotion of specific herbal products or brands.

Readers should exercise their discretion and judgment when applying the information from this book, and they are encouraged to conduct further research and seek guidance from healthcare professionals to make informed decisions about their health and well-being.

"Holistic Approaches to Managing Pancreatic Disorder" is a thorough and innovative resource that tackles the complex aspects of pancreatic health from an integrated and holistic perspective. The book begins with a detailed examination of the background, describing the anatomy and function of the pancreas, and then moves on to discuss the goal of the book, who the target audience is, what is covered, and how much is covered.

Chapter 1 takes the reader on a tour of pancreatic disorders, explaining the nuances of diseases like pancreatitis, pancreatic cancer, and diabetes mellitus. Chapter 2 then lays out a holistic perspective on health, defining holistic health and outlining the tenets of holistic healing. Chapter 2 then moves smoothly into the discussion of how holistic approaches are integrated with pancreatic health, falling under the purview of integrative medicine.

Chapters 3 through 6 thoroughly explain the critical role that diet, the mind-body connection, herbal remedies, and lifestyle modifications play in promoting pancreatic wellness.

The book summarizes many aspects of holistic care, ranging from dietary supplements, anti-inflammatory diets, and nutritional guidelines to stress's effect on pancreatic health and the promotion of mindfulness, meditation, yoga, acupuncture, and other lifestyle modifications.

Chapters 8 through 9 emphasize the value of patient empowerment and self-care, guiding readers on advocating for personal health, creating support networks, and offering useful resources like pancreatic-friendly recipes, meal plans, and cooking tips. Chapter 7 emphasizes collaborative care, and effective communication with healthcare providers, and substantiates its claims with compelling case studies showcasing successful integrative approaches.

With its systematic exploration of diverse dimensions, "Holistic Approaches to Managing Pancreatic Disorder" emerges not only as an indispensable guide for healthcare practitioners but also as an invaluable resource for patients seeking a comprehensive understanding and management of pancreatic disorders. Chapter 10 of the book culminates in a projection of pancreatic health, illuminating new trends in research, innovations, holistic therapies, and the evolving role of technology in pancreatic care.

Overview

Because of their complexity and potential severity, pancreatic disorders present significant challenges in the healthcare system. This book explores holistic approaches to managing pancreatic disorders, taking into account the many facets of these conditions. By looking at different aspects like medical, nutritional, psychological, and lifestyle factors, this all-encompassing approach aims to improve the overall care and well-being of people with pancreatic disorders.

Context

The study's backdrop is the growing incidence and impact of pancreatic disorders on world health. Disorders of the pancreas, such as pancreatitis and pancreatic cancer, pose complex diagnostic and therapeutic challenges. Because of the complex anatomy and physiology of the pancreas and the variety of etiological factors that lead to these disorders, a holistic understanding is necessary for effective management. This book provides a basis for the holistic approach it advocates by exploring the historical background of pancreatic research and the development of treatment modalities.

The Book's Objective

With a focus on medical advancements, nutritional interventions, psychological support, and lifestyle modifications, the book seeks to offer a nuanced perspective on addressing the complex needs of individuals with pancreatic conditions. Its goal goes beyond simple symptom management to foster a holistic understanding that takes into account the interplay of various factors influencing disease progression and patient outcomes.

The main goal of this book is to give healthcare professionals, researchers, and students a comprehensive resource that explores holistic strategies for managing pancreatic disorders.

Intended Audience

This book's intended readership is comprised of a broad spectrum of medical professionals, such as gastroenterologists, surgeons, oncologists, dietitians, psychologists, nurses, and students studying pancreatic disorders. It also serves researchers and students studying pancreatic disorders. By customizing content to meet the needs of various healthcare disciplines, the book hopes to promote interdisciplinary collaboration and promote a more integrative and holistic approach to pancreatic disorder management.

Range And Restraints

This book covers the full spectrum of managing pancreatic disorders, including medical, nutritional, psychological, and lifestyle aspects.

It also includes the most recent research findings, evidence-based practices, and emerging therapies pertinent to the field. That being said, it is important to recognize the limitations that come with any medical literature since healthcare is always changing and new information is always being added, some content may need to be updated; additionally, the book should not be used in place of personalized medical advice; instead, readers are encouraged to speak with healthcare providers for guidance tailored to their particular patient circumstances.

Holistic Methods Of Medicine

When it comes to medical management, a holistic approach to pancreatic disorders entails a comprehensive comprehension of the underlying pathophysiology as well as the integration of different medical interventions. This book delves into the most recent developments in the field, covering everything from pharmacological and surgical interventions to diagnostic modalities.

It also emphasizes personalized and targeted therapies, taking into account the heterogeneity of pancreatic disorders and the need for customized medical approaches for the best possible outcomes.

Dietary Tactics

Nutritional interventions are essential to the comprehensive management of pancreatic disorders. The book explores the complex relationship between diet and pancreatic health, taking into account the particular dietary needs of patients with pancreatitis or pancreatic cancer.

It offers evidence-based insights into optimizing nutritional interventions to support pancreatic function and reduce complications, as well as addressing issues like malabsorption and nutritional deficiencies that are frequently linked to pancreatic disorders.

Psychological Assistance

This section of the book explores the emotional and psychological impact of pancreatic conditions on patients and their families. It discusses strategies for coping with the mental health challenges associated with chronic diseases, including anxiety, depression, and coping with the uncertainty of prognosis. Support groups and psychotherapeutic interventions are incorporated into the discussion of coping strategies for individuals with pancreatic disorders. Although psychological well-being is often overlooked, it is essential to holistic care.

Changes In Lifestyle

This section of the book examines the effects of alcohol consumption, physical activity, stress, and smoking on pancreatic health and discusses strategies for lifestyle modifications aimed at preventing the onset of pancreatic disorders and supporting the management of existing conditions. From stress management techniques to smoking cessation programs, the book offers practical guidance on empowering individuals to make positive lifestyle changes for better pancreatic health. Lifestyle factors play a significant role in the development and progression of pancreatic disorders.

It is essential to manage pancreatic disorders holistically to fully address the complexity of these conditions. This book is an invaluable tool for researchers, students, and healthcare professionals as it provides comprehensive insights into the medical, nutritional, psychological, and lifestyle aspects of care. It also advocates for an integrative approach that goes beyond traditional disease-centric models. As the complexity of pancreatic disorders continues to be unveiled, adopting a holistic perspective will become increasingly important to improve patient outcomes and raise the standard of care in the field of pancreatic health.

CHAPTER ONE
UNDERSTANDING PANCREATIC DISORDERS

The pancreas is an essential organ that plays a multifaceted role in both endocrine and exocrine functions in the human body. Its complex anatomy consists of a head, body, and tail, and it is situated behind the stomach. Its main functions include secreting digestive enzymes into the small intestine and producing hormones like glucagon and insulin that control blood sugar levels. Because the pancreas is responsible for maintaining a delicate balance that is critical for overall health, understanding its anatomy and function is imperative.

Typical Pancreatic Conditions

Understanding the various forms of pancreatitis and their underlying causes is crucial for effective management and treatment. Pancreatic disorders can significantly impact the organ's normal functioning, leading to a variety of health complications. One common disorder is pancreatitis, which is characterized by inflammation of the pancreas. Pancreatitis can be acute or chronic, with symptoms ranging from nausea and abdominal pain to more severe complications.

Examining the complexities of pancreatic cancer, including risk factors, diagnostic techniques, and potential treatment modalities, is crucial for a thorough understanding of this debilitating disease. Pancreatic cancer is notorious for its aggressive nature and limited treatment options. It is frequently diagnosed at advanced stages, posing significant therapeutic challenges.

Because of its role in producing insulin, diabetes mellitus is a chronic metabolic disorder that is closely associated with the pancreas. Type 1 and type 2 diabetes both involve blood sugar dysregulation, which affects numerous organs and systems throughout the body. Developing a comprehensive strategy to manage diabetes is dependent on understanding the complex mechanisms and contributing factors, which can lead to more targeted interventions and better patient outcomes.

Integrated Methods For Treating Pancreatic Illnesses

A comprehensive understanding of the interrelated factors that contribute to the development and progression of pancreatic disorders is necessary for a holistic approach to management. It is imperative to integrate various disciplines, including gastroenterology, oncology, endocrinology, and surgery, for a well-rounded and successful approach to patient care.

When it comes to pancreatitis, holistic care involves not only treating acute episodes but also addressing underlying causes and risk factors. Dietary interventions, lifestyle changes, and ongoing monitoring for complications are all essential parts of a holistic approach. Working together with other medical professionals, such as mental health and nutritionists, can further improve the overall quality of life for those who suffer from pancreatitis.

Because pancreatic cancer is so complex, managing it calls for a multidisciplinary approach. Conventional treatment modalities include surgery, chemotherapy, and radiation therapy; however, a holistic approach goes beyond these measures. Pain management, psychosocial support, and supportive care are critical components of enhancing the quality of life for patients with pancreatic cancer. Furthermore, ongoing research into targeted therapies and immunotherapies holds promise for more individualized and successful treatments.

The comprehensive management of diabetes mellitus requires not only glucose control but also lifestyle modifications, patient education, and psychological well-being. Since the pancreas plays a crucial role in insulin production, a detailed understanding of the disease is necessary to customize interventions for each patient. Endocrinologists, dietitians, and mental health professionals must work together to ensure comprehensive diabetes management. Technological innovations, like insulin pumps and continuous glucose monitoring, further enhance this patient-centered and integrated approach.

a comprehensive understanding of the complex interactions that exist between the pancreas and general health is necessary for a holistic approach to managing pancreatic disorders. By addressing the anatomical, physiological, and pathological aspects of the pancreas, healthcare professionals can create more effective strategies for early detection, prevention, and treatment of pancreatic disorders. This integrative approach not only improves patient outcomes but also raises the quality of life for those who are dealing with these difficult conditions.

CHAPTER TWO
HOLISTIC APPROACH TO HEALTH

In managing pancreatic disorders, a holistic approach acknowledges that the health of the pancreas is not isolated but is intricately linked to overall well-being. This paradigm shift from focusing solely on symptomatic treatment to addressing the root causes of ailments is integral to holistic health. Generally speaking, a holistic approach to health emphasizes the interconnectedness of various aspects of an individual's well-being, considering physical, mental, emotional, and spiritual dimensions.

What Is Meant By Holistic Health?

In the context of pancreatic disorders, a holistic definition would involve understanding the pancreas not only as an isolated organ but as part of a larger network that includes lifestyle, nutrition, mental health, and environmental factors. This broader perspective enables healthcare practitioners to develop interventions that promote overall health and prevent the recurrence of pancreatic disorders. Holistic health is a multidimensional concept that encompasses the entire spectrum of an individual's life and goes beyond the absence of disease.

Fundamentals Of Integrative Medicine

In the context of pancreatic disorders, these principles guide healthcare practitioners to explore therapeutic modalities beyond conventional medicine. Personalized care, consideration of the mind-body connection, emphasis on prevention, and the integration of various healing modalities, such as nutrition, exercise, and stress management, are common holistic healing principles. These beliefs are at the core of the holistic healing philosophy, which holds that the body has an innate capacity for self-healing and that interventions should support and enhance this natural process.

Pancreatic Health With Integrative Medicine

A more patient-centered and holistic approach to managing pancreatic disorders is fostered by the concept of integrative medicine, which is the blending of conventional and alternative approaches to healthcare. In the context of pancreatic health, integrative medicine combines traditional medical treatments with complementary therapies, emphasizing the value of addressing the whole person rather than just the disease. Integrative approaches may include dietary changes, acupuncture, yoga, and mindfulness practices, all of which are tailored to support pancreatic health.

Together, these ideas support a more comprehensive approach to managing pancreatic disorders by highlighting a move away from a narrow focus on managing symptoms and toward a more comprehensive consideration of the individual's overall well-being. We will go into more detail about each of these ideas in the sections that follow to give you a more thorough understanding of their implications for pancreatic health.

A Holistic Perspective On Health

A holistic approach to health is a paradigm that goes beyond the conventional biomedical model and acknowledges the complex interactions between different elements that contribute to an individual's well-being. The pancreas, being an essential organ in the digestive and endocrine systems, is a key player in preserving homeostasis within the body. Pancreatic health from a holistic standpoint recognizes the significant influences of stress, nutrition, lifestyle, and emotional health on pancreatic function. By taking these interrelated factors into account, medical professionals can create more complex and efficacious plans for treating pancreatic disorders.

What Is Meant By Holistic Health?

A holistic definition of pancreatic health takes into account factors like mental and emotional states, social interactions, and environmental influences. It goes beyond a reductionist view of health and recognizes that the body is a complex system where each part influences and is influenced by the whole. In the context of pancreatic disorders, holistic health entails an understanding that the health of the pancreas is closely linked to the overall health of the individual. This comprehensive understanding helps healthcare professionals design interventions that not only target pancreatic disorders but also promote holistic well-being.

Fundamentals Of Integrative Medicine

Personalized care is another important principle, acknowledging that each individual is unique and may respond differently to interventions. By taking into consideration the mind-body connection, holistic healing principles emphasize the impact of mental and emotional states on physical health, urging a more comprehensive approach to managing pancreatic disorders. The beliefs that underpin the concept of addressing health in its entirety are summarized as follows personalized care is the belief that the body has an innate ability to heal itself.

Pancreatic Health With Integrative Medicine

When it comes to pancreatic health, integrative medicine is a synergistic approach that blends traditional medical treatments with complementary therapies. It recognizes the limitations of a purely biomedical approach and looks for alternative ways to support the pancreas and the individual's overall health. Integrative medicine encompasses a range of modalities, such as nutritional interventions, acupuncture, herbal medicine, and mind-body practices like yoga and meditation. By combining these complementary approaches, medical professionals hope to improve the efficacy of conventional treatments and address the complex nature of pancreatic disorders.

the holistic approach to managing pancreatic disorders entails acknowledging the interdependence of different facets of health and well-being. By adopting an integrative medicine perspective, defining pancreatic health holistically, and comprehending the tenets of holistic healing, medical professionals can create more comprehensive and successful treatment plans for pancreatic disorders that not only address symptoms but also foster overall well-being and encourage a move toward a patient-centered and integrative healthcare model.

CHAPTER THREE
NUTRITION AND PANCREATIC HEALTH

The role that nutrition plays in maintaining the overall health of the pancreas cannot be overstated. Disorders of the pancreas, like pancreatitis and pancreatic cancer, frequently result in impaired nutritional absorption and digestive function. Appropriate nutrition becomes critical for symptom relief, treatment support, and overall quality of life improvement for those who suffer from these conditions.

Nutritional interventions are critical not only in the acute stages of pancreatic disorders but also in their long-term management to prevent complications and promote optimal pancreatic health.

Dietary Recommendations For The Health Of The Pancreas

Following particular dietary guidelines is essential when it comes to managing pancreatic disorders because they present special challenges.

 One of the main pillars of nutritional management for pancreatic disorders is an anti-inflammatory diet. Since chronic inflammation is a common feature of many pancreatic diseases, following an anti-inflammatory diet can help reduce inflammation, relieve symptoms, and improve the patient's overall health. Pro-inflammatory foods include processed sugars, saturated fats, and refined carbohydrates.

Furthermore, a key component of maintaining pancreatic health is incorporating nutrient-rich foods. These foods are high in vital vitamins, minerals, and antioxidants that support pancreatic function.

Fruits, vegetables, whole grains, and lean proteins are some of the main ingredients of a nutrient-rich diet for pancreatic health.

By giving priority to these food sources, people can make sure their bodies are getting the nutrients they need to support pancreatic function and help in the healing process.

Dietary supplements are a vital component of the holistic approach to managing pancreatic disorders. Patients may find it difficult to receive enough nutrients from their diet alone due to the potential malabsorption issues associated with these conditions; in these cases, supplements can fill the nutritional gap by offering essential vitamins and minerals in a concentrated form.

For example, pancreatic enzyme supplements can help with the digestion and absorption of nutrients, making up for the impaired pancreatic function and promoting better overall nutritional status.

Finally, dietary recommendations for pancreatic health are based on a multimodal strategy that targets inflammation, emphasizes foods high in nutrients, and includes dietary supplements.

This comprehensive approach seeks to both treat acute phases of the disease's symptoms and lay the groundwork for long-term pancreatic health.

CHAPTER FOUR
LINK BETWEEN MIND AND BODY

The integration of stress management strategies into the holistic approach to pancreatic disorders is necessary because the interplay between the mind and body is complex and often emphasized by the impact of stress on pancreatic health. Stress, both acute and chronic, is a significant factor in the development and exacerbation of pancreatic disorders. Since the pancreas is an important organ in the endocrine and digestive systems, it is vulnerable to the influence of stress hormones, especially cortisol. Chronic stress may contribute to inflammation and oxidative stress in the pancreas, potentially increasing the risk of pancreatic disorders like pancreatitis.

In the context of pancreatic disorders, mindfulness may be a useful tool to mitigate stress-induced inflammation and promote a more balanced physiological state. Additionally, meditation, which includes a variety of techniques like focused attention and loving-kindness meditation, has demonstrated positive effects on stress reduction and psychological resilience. Mindfulness, which has its roots in ancient contemplative practices, involves cultivating awareness of the present moment without judgment. Previous studies have indicated the potential of mindfulness-based interventions in reducing stress levels and enhancing emotional regulation.

As a holistic mind-body practice, yoga has the potential to support pancreatic health and manage pancreatic disorders. It consists of physical postures, or asanas, breath control, or pranayama, and meditation. Some yoga postures are thought to stimulate the pancreas and improve its function from a physiological standpoint. Additionally, the focus on controlled breathing in pranayama practices may have a positive effect on stress reduction and the autonomic nervous system, which is involved in pancreatic function.

Finally, the holistic aspect of yoga goes beyond physical exercise, encompassing mental and emotional well-being. Regular yoga practice has been linked to lower stress levels, improved mood, and improved quality of life.

the mind-body connection is essential to the holistic management of pancreatic disorders.

The impact of stress on pancreatic health emphasizes the need to implement stress management strategies. Mindfulness and meditation, with their research-proven benefits in stress reduction and emotional regulation, are useful tools for enhancing overall well-being. Additionally, the holistic practice of yoga, which includes physical postures, breath control, and meditation, presents a comprehensive approach to improving pancreatic health. Healthcare providers can adopt a holistic perspective by incorporating these ideas into the management of pancreatic disorders.

CHAPTER FIVE
HERBAL REMEDIES AND ADVANCED THERAPIES

The comprehensive treatment of pancreatic disorders involves a variety of approaches that extend beyond traditional medical interventions. Among these approaches is the use of herbal remedies and alternative therapies.

Herbal supplements have garnered interest recently due to their potential role in promoting pancreatic health. Traditional medicine has long utilized herbs like aloe vera, turmeric, and ginger, which have been studied for their antioxidant and anti-inflammatory properties. These properties are especially pertinent when it comes to pancreatic disorders, as disease progression is largely dependent on inflammation and oxidative stress.

Both Acupressure And Acupuncture

Traditional Chinese medicine gave rise to alternative therapeutic modalities such as acupressure and acupuncture, which stimulate specific body pressure points or acupuncture points to restore the flow of energy or Qi. In the context of pancreatic health, acupuncture has been studied for its ability to reduce inflammation and pain associated with conditions such as pancreatitis, and acupressure, a non-invasive variation of acupuncture, has been studied as a complementary approach to improve overall well-being and alleviate symptoms in people with pancreatic disorders. While the scientific community has been able to identify the mechanisms underlying the effects of a cup

Pancreatic Disorders And Homeopathy

Another component of holistic management for pancreatic disorders is homeopathy, an alternative medicine system based on the idea that "like cures like." In homeopathic treatment, highly diluted substances that would cause similar symptoms in a healthy person are administered to stimulate the body's self-healing mechanisms.

Although homeopathy has been more frequently linked to chronic conditions, its use as a complementary strategy in pancreatic disorders has been investigated. Homeopathic remedies customized to each patient's unique symptoms and constitutional factors seek to address the underlying imbalances that contribute to pancreatic dysfunction; however, opinions in the scientific community regarding homeopathy's effectiveness remain divided, with little high-quality evidence the holistic management of pancreatic disorders encompasses a diverse range of approaches, including herbal remedies, acupuncture, acupressure, and homeopathy. These alternative therapies strive to address the multifaceted nature of pancreatic disorders by targeting symptoms, reducing inflammation, and promoting overall well-being. While some studies suggest potential benefits, it is crucial to acknowledge the current limitations in scientific evidence and the need for further research to establish the efficacy and safety of these approaches. Integrating alternative therapies into the comprehensive care of individuals with pancreatic disorders requires careful consideration of patient preferences, individualized treatment plans, and collaboration between conventional and alternative healthcare providers. As the field continues to evolve, a balanced and evidence-based approach will contribute to the development of holistic strategies that optimize the well-being of individuals with pancreatic disorders.

CHAPTER SIX
MODIFICATIONS TO LIFESTYLE FOR PANCREATIC HEALTH

A comprehensive strategy for managing pancreatic disorders entails addressing a person's lifestyle to promote overall health and well-being.

One important component of this strategy is the regular integration of physical activity and exercise into daily routines. Exercise is essential for maintaining a healthy weight, lowering inflammation, and enhancing insulin sensitivity—all of which are important factors in pancreatic health. Studies have demonstrated the beneficial effects of both aerobic and resistance training exercises on the pancreas, which in turn improves blood sugar regulation and overall metabolic function. Additionally, exercise can improve circulation, guaranteeing that the pancreas gets enough blood flow to support its optimal functioning.

Adopting good sleep hygiene practices, such as maintaining a consistent sleep schedule, creating a comfortable sleep environment, and avoiding stimulants before bedtime, is crucial for promoting pancreatic wellness. Sleep deprivation and irregular sleep schedules may lead to insulin resistance, a key factor in the development of pancreatic disorders. Quality sleep is integral to overall health, and disruptions in sleep patterns can have adverse effects on metabolic processes, including those related to pancreatic function.

To manage pancreatic disorders holistically, quitting smoking is crucial. Smoking is a significant risk factor for the onset and progression of pancreatic diseases, including pancreatic cancer. The chemicals in tobacco smoke can cause inflammation, oxidative stress, and damage to pancreatic cells. By kicking the habit, people can lessen these negative effects, which lowers their risk of developing pancreatic disorders and improves their overall health.

Additionally, quitting smoking improves their cardiovascular health, which further supports the holistic well-being of those who are at risk for or already have pancreatic disorders.

incorporating these lifestyle modifications into a comprehensive management plan can greatly improve the general health and well-being of people with or at risk for pancreatic disorders. Exercise and physical activity are important for weight management, insulin sensitivity, and overall metabolic health. Sleep hygiene is critical for preserving optimal metabolic function.

Finally, quitting smoking is critical for preventing the damaging effects of tobacco smoke on the pancreas.

Nutritional Strategies For Pancreatic Health

Because nutrition has a significant impact on pancreatic health, a holistic approach to addressing pancreatic problems includes dietary treatments. The next paragraphs discuss particular dietary modifications that can improve pancreatic well-being.

In the context of pancreatic health, the importance of eating a well-balanced and nutrient-dense diet cannot be emphasized. Eating a diet high in fruits, vegetables, whole grains, and lean proteins supplies vital nutrients that support the pancreas's proper functioning. Foods high in antioxidants, like nuts, berries, and green leafy vegetables, help combat oxidative stress, which is linked to the development of pancreatic disorders. Additionally, eating a diet high in fiber helps with digestion and can help with blood sugar regulation, which lessens the load on the pancreas.

Maintaining a balanced omega-3 to omega-6 fatty acid ratio is essential for reducing inflammation and promoting overall metabolic well-being. Moderation of fat intake, especially that of saturated and trans fats, is another important dietary consideration. High-fat diets can contribute to obesity and insulin resistance, both of which are risk factors for pancreatic disorders. Pancreatic health can be supported by choosing healthy fats like those found in avocados, olive oil, and fatty fish while limiting the intake of processed and fried foods.

When it comes to pancreatic disorders, certain dietary factors need to be taken into account.

For example, pancreatic enzyme insufficiency needs to be managed. People who suffer from conditions such as chronic pancreatitis might need to take supplements that help them digest nutrients. Working with healthcare providers, such as dietitians, to customize diet plans for each patient is an essential part of managing pancreatic disorders holistically.

A comprehensive approach to supporting pancreatic health involves addressing specific dietary needs based on individual conditions, addressing fat intake, highlighting antioxidant-rich foods, and adopting a nutritious and well-balanced diet.

Emotional Regulation And Stress Handling In Pancreatic Health

The importance of stress reduction techniques and emotional well-being in promoting pancreatic health is explored in the following paragraphs. Chronic stress has been linked to adverse effects on the pancreas, including inflammation and impaired insulin function. Therefore, addressing stress management and emotional well-being is crucial in the holistic management of pancreatic disorders.

Stress reduction techniques, such as mindfulness meditation, deep breathing exercises, and yoga, can help lessen the negative effects of stress on the pancreas.

People who are at risk for pancreatic disorders or who are already experiencing them should practice stress management because long-term exposure to elevated cortisol levels can cause insulin resistance and inflammation, two conditions that are detrimental to pancreatic health.

A holistic approach to managing pancreatic disorders can benefit from addressing mental health concerns through counseling, therapy, or support groups. Additionally, cultivating a positive and supportive social environment can have a beneficial impact on emotional well-being, further supporting pancreatic health. Pancreatic health is also significantly influenced by emotional well-being, with conditions like depression and anxiety linked to an increased risk of pancreatic disorders.

The relationship between emotional stress and pancreatic function is a prime example of the mind-body connection.

Mindfulness-based stress reduction programs have demonstrated promise in lowering inflammation and increasing insulin sensitivity, further demonstrating the connection between mental and physical health. Including these practices in the overall management plan for pancreatic disorders is crucial for a comprehensive and all-encompassing approach.

a comprehensive approach to managing pancreatic disorders must include stress management and emotional well-being. Reducing chronic stress and taking care of mental health issues are important ways to improve pancreatic health and well-being. Understanding the complex relationship between the mind and the pancreas emphasizes the significance of a holistic approach that takes into account both physical and emotional aspects of health.

CHAPTER SEVEN
INTEGRATING CONVENTIONAL AND HOLISTIC APPROACHES

The multifaceted nature of pancreatic disorders makes a comprehensive and integrative approach necessary for effective management. One promising strategy to address this complexity is the integration of conventional and holistic approaches. Conventional medicine emphasizes pharmacological interventions and surgical procedures, but holistic approaches that take into account the patient's overall well-being and include lifestyle modifications, nutritional support, and alternative therapies can be added. This integration aims to provide a more individualized and patient-centric approach to managing pancreatic disorders, optimizing treatment outcomes, and enhancing the quality of life for affected individuals.

Cooperative Healthcare

As a leader in the comprehensive management of pancreatic disorders, collaborative care highlights the value of a multidisciplinary healthcare team. In this setting, medical professionals from different specialties—such as nutritionists, pain specialists, gastroenterologists, and practitioners of alternative medicine—work together to develop a comprehensive and customized treatment plan. Through encouraging communication and cooperation between different specialists, collaborative care tackles the intricate interplay of physical, psychological, and social factors related to pancreatic disorders. This method not only guarantees a more thorough understanding of the patient's condition but also makes it easier to implement a customized and synergistic treatment strategy, promoting holistic care.

Interacting With Healthcare Professionals

A key component of successful pancreatic disorder management is effective communication between healthcare providers and patients. Practitioners should have honest and open discussions with patients, developing a relationship based on mutual trust and understanding. When it comes to holistic approaches, this communication goes beyond simply exchanging medical information and includes conversations about dietary changes, lifestyle modifications, and the integration of alternative therapies. Patients should be involved in their care, and healthcare providers should pay close attention to their concerns, preferences, and experiences. This collaborative communication model allows for the development of a shared decision-making process, empowering patients.

Case Studies Effective Integrative Methodologies

Healthcare professionals can gain a deeper understanding of the practical implementation and potential benefits of holistic care by examining case studies that highlight successful integrative approaches to managing pancreatic disorders. These case studies also highlight the importance of tailoring interventions to individual patient needs, emphasizing the uniqueness of each case and the necessity of a personalized, patient-centric approach in the holistic management process. The integration of conventional and holistic modalities can lead to improved patient outcomes, and these cases serve as illustrative examples of how this can be achieved.

Integrating conventional and holistic approaches presents a promising paradigm for the management of pancreatic disorders. Collaborative care emphasizes a multidisciplinary healthcare team, offering a comprehensive and holistic perspective.

To build trust and enable shared decision-making within the holistic framework, effective communication between patients and healthcare providers is crucial. Analyzing case studies that highlight successful integrative approaches provides practical insights into the real-world application of these strategies, highlighting the significance of personalized, patient-centric care in optimizing outcomes for individuals with pancreatic disorders.

CHAPTER EIGHT
SELF-CARE AND PATIENT EMPOWERMENT

Advocating for personal health becomes a cornerstone in this approach, emphasizing the importance of patient engagement and education. Pancreatic disorders, which include a range of conditions such as pancreatitis and pancreatic cancer, pose significant challenges to patients and healthcare providers alike. A holistic approach to managing pancreatic disorders involves empowering patients through active participation in their healthcare journey and promoting self-care strategies.

Promoting Individual Health

Encouraging patients to ask questions, seek clarification, and actively participate in decision-making processes fosters a sense of ownership over their well-being.

Providing patients with comprehensive education on the nature of pancreatic disorders, treatment options, and lifestyle modifications is essential to empowering them to take charge of their health. Healthcare providers play a pivotal role in ensuring that patients understand the complexities of their condition, including the causes, risk factors, and potential complications.

In addition, promoting a healthy lifestyle becomes critical when advocating for personal health. Individuals with pancreatic disorders can benefit from dietary modifications, like a low-fat diet, and lifestyle changes, like regular exercise.

These changes not only improve general well-being but can also have a positive impact on the disorder's progression. Ultimately, advocating for personal health highlights the partnership between patients and healthcare providers in making decisions that improve quality of life.

Putting Together A Support Network

Understanding the psychological and emotional effects of pancreatic disorders, the holistic approach includes creating a strong support network for patients. A support network is made up of friends, family, healthcare providers, and patient support groups.

These groups work together to support patients' emotional health and enable them to deal with the difficulties posed by their condition.

Building a strong support system guarantees that patients feel understood, valued, and better able to cope with the complexities of pancreatic disorders. Family members and friends play a crucial role in providing practical assistance, emotional support, and encouragement.

In-person or online patient support groups offer a platform for individuals facing similar challenges to share experiences, insights, and coping strategies.

Healthcare providers, as part of the support system, should prioritize open communication and empathy, addressing not only the physical symptoms but also the emotional aspects of the illness.

Keeping An Eye On And Controlling Symptoms At Home

A key component of a comprehensive strategy for managing pancreatic disorders is equipping patients with the knowledge and abilities to keep an eye on and control their symptoms at home. This includes teaching patients how to spot early warning indicators, why changes in symptoms are important, and how to effectively assess themselves.

The ability to identify and promptly report symptoms enables patients to take an active role in their ongoing care, facilitating timely interventions and preventing potential complications. Healthcare providers should also educate patients on how to use monitoring devices, if applicable, such as blood glucose meters for those with diabetes-related pancreatic issues. Patients should be empowered to monitor key indicators, such as pain levels, digestive issues, and appetite changes.

In addition, home symptom management involves lifestyle changes and self-care routines.

Patients should receive education on pain management methods, dietary changes, and stress-reduction tactics. This comprehensive approach guarantees that patients have the resources and know-how to deal with day-to-day difficulties related to pancreatic disorders, thereby encouraging a sense of control over their health.

Ultimately, the goal of the holistic approach to managing pancreatic disorders through patient empowerment and self-care is to improve the overall quality of life for people with pancreatic disorders by addressing the physical aspects of the illness, acknowledging the significance of emotional well-being, and empowering patients to monitor and manage their symptoms at home. This comprehensive strategy involves advocating for personal health, establishing a support system, and empowering patients to monitor and manage their symptoms at home.

CHAPTER NINE
MEAL PLANS AND RECIPES

Pancreatic disorders, which include a variety of conditions like pancreatitis and pancreatic cancer, require a comprehensive and all-encompassing approach to management. Within this framework, dietary considerations are critical to symptom relief, healing, and improving pancreatic health overall. One aspect of this approach is the creation and use of pancreatic-friendly recipes that are customized to meet the unique dietary requirements and restrictions associated with pancreatic disorders.

1 Recipes Suitable for Pancreas

Creating recipes that are pancreas-friendly requires a careful selection of ingredients that are low in fat, easy to digest, and high in essential nutrients. Lean proteins, like chicken and fish, as well as carbohydrates from whole grains and fibrous fruits and vegetables, can be included in these recipes. Plant-based oils containing omega-3 fatty acids can also be helpful. Reducing the amount of saturated fats and refined sugars can also be extremely important. Developing a variety of tasty recipes guarantees that people with pancreatic disorders have a variety of options to suit their tastes while adhering to strict dietary restrictions.

2 Example Menus

The process of creating sample meal plans entails incorporating pancreatic-friendly recipes into a well-balanced daily diet. Oatmeal with fresh berries and a lean protein source, like Greek yogurt, can be eaten for breakfast. A quinoa salad with leafy greens, vegetables, and grilled chicken can be eaten for lunch to supply necessary nutrients without overloading the digestive system. Baked fish with steamed vegetables and a side of whole-grain rice can be eaten for dinner. Snacks can include tiny amounts of nuts, seeds, or fruit to sustain energy levels in between meals.

Water infusion with citrus fruits can be a refreshing and pancreas-friendly beverage. These sample meal plans not only address nutritional requirements but also focus on the frequency and distribution of

Recipe Advice For Healthy Pancreas

Cooking for pancreatic health means using certain techniques to keep food nutritious while making it easier to digest. Baking, steaming, and grilling are better than frying because they lower the total fat content of meals. Herbs and spices can add flavor without using too much salt or fat. Portion control is also important because eating smaller, more frequent meals can help manage pancreatic workload. Food preparation techniques like chopping and blending can be used to create textures that are easier to digest, especially for people who have trouble chewing or swallowing. Finally, adding foods high in probiotics, like yogurt with live cultures, may support gut health.

It is possible to mitigate symptoms, support healing, and enhance overall well-being by customizing dietary choices to accommodate the unique needs of individuals with pancreatic disorders. This integrative approach not only addresses the nutritional aspects of pancreatic health but also takes into account the practical aspects of meal preparation and consumption, offering a comprehensive framework for individuals seeking to manage pancreatic disorders effectively. In conclusion, a holistic approach to managing pancreatic disorders involves a multifaceted strategy that includes the development of pancreatic-friendly recipes, sample meal plans, and cooking tips for optimal pancreatic health.

CHAPTER TEN
PROSPECTS FOR PANCREATIC HEALTH IN THE FUTURE
Investigations And Novelties

The field of pancreatic health is continually changing due to discoveries and ongoing research. Scientists and medical professionals are exploring the complex mechanisms that underlie pancreatic disorders to find novel approaches to prevent, diagnose, and treat these conditions.

Additionally, the development of advanced imaging techniques, proteomics, and genomics has allowed for a deeper understanding of pancreatic diseases at the molecular level and has made it possible to identify genetic markers, which opens the door to personalized medicine approaches that are customized for individual patients. Finally, ongoing clinical trials are investigating novel pharmaceutical interventions and therapeutic modalities, providing hope for more efficient and

New Trends In Holistic Medicine

Integrative medicine, which combines conventional and alternative therapies, is becoming more common. It emphasizes a patient-centered approach to care. Holistic approaches to managing pancreatic disorders are becoming more and more popular as a complementary aspect of conventional medical interventions.

 Beyond pharmacological treatments, holistic therapies encompass a wide range of practices that consider the interconnectedness of physical, mental, and emotional well-being.

Nutritional interventions, including specialized diets and supplements, are being explored for their potential to support pancreatic health. Mind-body practices, like meditation and yoga, are becoming more widely recognized for their role in stress reduction, which is crucial given the established links between chronic stress and pancreatic disorders.

Technology's Place In Pancreatic Care

Innovations in imaging technologies, like magnetic resonance imaging (MRI) and endoscopic ultrasound, offer comprehensive views of the anatomy and physiology of the pancreas, facilitating early detection and precise diagnosis. The use of robotics-assisted surgery is growing in precision and minimally invasive procedures, resulting in shorter recovery times for patients and better overall outcomes.

Telemedicine is enabling remote consultations and monitoring, improving accessibility to healthcare services, particularly for those living in remote areas. Wearable devices and mobile applications are being developed to empower patients in self-monitoring and managing their pancreas.

CONCLUSION
Summary Of The Main Ideas

In conclusion, research, holistic therapies, and technological advancements will all dynamically interact to shape pancreatic health in the future. Research is revealing the molecular details of pancreatic disorders, opening the door to personalized medicine and targeted interventions. Holistic therapies, which include mind-body practices and nutritional approaches, are becoming more widely recognized for their ability to promote overall well-being and supplement traditional medical treatments.

Technology is reshaping pancreatic care through telemedicine, wearables, robotic-assisted surgery, and advanced imaging. These developments will result in a more integrated and patient-centered healthcare environment.

Motivation For A Holistic Lifestyle

A growing number of people are recognizing that holistic living is a fundamental component of well-being as we navigate the changing landscape of pancreatic health. People are being encouraged to adopt holistic lifestyles by encouraging healthy habits related to nutrition and mental health. Nutritional education and awareness campaigns can empower people to make decisions that support pancreatic health.

Additionally, cultivating a culture of mindfulness and stress management can help lower the risk of pancreatic disorders. Adopting a holistic approach involves not only addressing current health issues but also emphasizing preventive measures and proactive self-care. By incorporating holistic living into daily practices, people can improve their overall health and well-being.